FERMENTED VEGETABLES

Top 30 Delicious Recipes for Fermented Vegetables and Probiotic Foods that will Restore your Optimal Gut Health

The Gut Repair Book Series, Book 3

BY

SARAH JONES

© Copyright 2017 by Sarah Jones - All rights reserved.

This document is geared towards providing exact and reliable information in regards to the topic and issue covered. The publication is sold with the idea that the publisher is not required to render accounting, officially permitted, or otherwise, qualified services. If advice is necessary, legal or professional, a practiced individual in the profession should be ordered.

From a Declaration of Principles which was accepted and approved equally by a Committee of the American Bar Association and a Committee of Publishers and Associations.

In no way is it legal to reproduce, duplicate, or transmit any part of this document in either electronic means or in printed format. Recording of this publication is strictly prohibited and any storage of this document is not allowed unless with written permission from the publisher. All rights reserved.

The information provided herein is stated to be truthful and consistent, in that any liability, in terms of inattention or otherwise, by any usage or abuse of any policies, processes, or directions contained within is the solitary and utter responsibility of the recipient reader. Under no circumstances will any legal responsibility or blame be held against the publisher for any reparation, damages, or monetary loss due to the information herein, either directly or indirectly.

Respective authors own all copyrights not held by the publisher.

The information herein is offered for informational purposes solely, and is universal as so. The presentation of the information is without contract or any type of guarantee assurance.

The trademarks that are used are without any consent, and the publication of the trademark is without permission or backing by the trademark owner. All trademarks and brands within this book are for clarifying purposes only and are the owned by the owners themselves, not affiliated with this document.

Table of Contents

Introduction 1

Chapter 1 – The Wonderful Benefits of Probiotics 2

Chapter 2 – Setting Up a Probiotic-Friendly Kitchen 11

Chapter 3 – Choosing the Best Ingredients 21

Chapter 4 – Fermented Vegetable Recipes 25

    Classic Sauerkraut 25

    Blaukraut 27

    Gingered Carrot Kraut 29

    Celeriac Kraut 31

    Cauliflower Kraut 33

    Zesty Lemon Kraut 35

    Zesty Spinach Kraut 37

    Curtido Rojo 39

    Basic Pickled Cucumbers 42

    Pickled Asparagus 44

    Napa Cabbage Kimchi 46

    Arugula Kimchi 49

    Southern Fermented Coleslaw 51

    Spicy Brussels Sprouts Pickles 54

    Pickled Carrot Sticks 56

    Vietnamese Daikon and Carrot Pickles 58

    Japanese Pickled Cabbage 60

    Coriander Pickles 62

    Spiced Cherry Tomato Pickles 63

    Shiitake Mushroom Pickles 65

    Spicy Mexican-Style Pickles 67

    Celery Relish 69

    Fermented Cilantro 71

    Spiced Collard Green Relish 73

    Sweet Corn Relish 75

    Fermented Eggplant 77

    Garlic Paste 79

    Prepared Horseradish 80

    Onion Relish 81

Chapter 5 – Other Probiotic Food Recipes 83

    Cinnamon Lemon and Lime Preserves 83

    Peach and Lime Chutney 85

    Apple Curry Chutney 87

    Hummus 89

    Ginger Ale 91

    Kombucha 93

    Basic Yogurt 95

    Kefir 97

Conclusion 98

Introduction

The thought of making sauerkraut, kimchi, pickles, and other probiotic foods at home might sound intimidating. However, with the right guide, anyone can become an expert!

In this book, you will learn about the importance of probiotics in your diet. You will also learn of the benefits of eating fermented vegetables aside from probiotics. In addition, you will find a quick and easy guide on how to set up an ideal kitchen for fermenting vegetables and how to find the best ingredients. Most importantly, you will acquire over 30 easy recipes for a wide variety of fermented vegetables and other probiotic foods.

Having a strong immune system is one of the greatest assets anyone can ever have, which is why it is essential for everyone to eat probiotic foods every day. The best way to make this a sustainable part of the diet is to make fermented vegetables and probiotic foods yourself, that's why I would now like to invite you to turn to chapter I to start your journey towards healthy digestive and immune system.

Chapter 1 – The Wonderful Benefits of Probiotics

By choosing this book, there is a high chance you are already familiar with the topic of probiotics, especially if you are fond of researching about health and fitness. However, if the topic is relatively new to you, then this chapter will explain to you the nature and purpose of probiotics as it relates to your health.

Probiotics, strictly speaking, refers to the beneficial bacteria present in the intestinal tract of all healthy mammals, including humans. They are usually called probiotic bacteria, although many also refer to them as probiotic flora or probiotic microflora because they are often considered as part of the plant kingdom.

Nevertheless, maintaining a healthy balance of probiotics inside your gut is good for you because of many reasons, one of which is that they protect you from the harmful bacteria present in your surroundings, including the foods you eat.

For instance, think about the last thing you ate today. Can you guarantee that it does not contain anything harmful? No one can because no matter how well we prepare our food, it is never a hundred percent microbe-free. In fact, most of the foods we eat contain microbes, toxins, and chemicals, especially if they are processed foods or foods not prepared in a sanitary environment.

As soon as the food is in the intestinal tract, a battle of microbes ensues – on your side are the probiotics or the healthy bacteria, such as *Lactobacilli* and *Bifidobacteria*. Behind the enemy lines are all the harmful microbes that are attempting to invade your body, such as *Candida albicans* and *E. coli*.

The stronger the probiotics are inside your gut, the better they are at inhibiting the growth of the pathogens. On the other hand, if the probiotics in your intestinal tract is insufficient or weak, then it is only natural for the pathogens to overcome them.

How Probiotics Take Action

To this day, scientists are still conducting further research on how probiotics work in the body, and how they create a barrier against harmful microbes. So far, they have come up with a number of scientifically proven explanations.

One explanation is that there is a competition for receptor sites between certain probiotics and the harmful bacteria. As soon as both enter the intestinal tract, both will fight each other to attach to the receptor sites found in the epithelial cells making up the intestinal lining. Keep in mind that epithelial cells not only make up the intestinal lining, but also in all the membranous tissues that cover the internal organs of the body, including the inside of the mouth and the vagina.

As soon as the probiotics are attached to the receptor sites, a reaction on the latter takes place. What happens is the epithelial cells will start to produce the mucus that serve as protection against the pathogens. Thus, the harmful microbes can no longer adhere to the receptor sites and the potential harm they could have caused had they been able to. Unfortunately, if there is not enough probiotics in your body to get to the receptor sites then the pathogens can gain access to them. This will lead to the colonization of harmful bacteria that will then lead to the development of a disease.

Another explanation as to how probiotics benefit the body is their positive impact on the immune system. One way through which they do this is stimulating the immune cells to secrete certain protein molecules called cytokines and antibodies. The role of these molecules is to regulate the immune system and promote healthy inflammation in response to any harmful pathogens that enter the body.

That said, the largest mass of immune cells in the entire body is found in the intestinal tract and it is called "gut-associated lymphoid tissue" or GALT. Cytokines cause the intestinal lining to be less permeable to toxins and harmful microbes while antibodies identify and neutralize the antigens, or any substance that the body recognizes as a threat.

Unfortunately, if there is not enough probiotics in the GALT to stimulate the secretion of these protein molecules then it is all too easy for pathogens to enter the bloodstream. Aside from GALT, immune cells can also be found in places where they are most needed, such as the spleen, the lungs, and the tonsils.

Aside from these two functions of blocking receptor sites from harmful microbes and stimulating the immune cells to produce protective protein molecules, certain probiotic strains also serve a third important function – to help prevent an autoimmune response and minimize the effects of anaphylaxis and asthma.

Scientists are still looking for a better explanation on how exactly they can do this, but the general theory is that probiotic bacteria help the immune cells become better at their job of recognizing which antigens are harmful pathogens (such as salmonella E. coli) and which ones are not.

For instance, some people are highly allergic to peanuts even though they do not necessarily contain anything that is truly "harmful" to the body. Yet if the person allergic to them will accidentally consume them, the immune system will go on hyperdrive and trigger inflammation not only in the intestinal tract, but also in all other areas where immune cells are present. This can potentially lead to anaphylactic shock, or the rapid and potentially fatal hypersensitive reaction to an antigen.

A healthy balance of probiotics can minimize the effects of such a predicament. While this does not mean a person who is allergic to peanuts can freely eat them once he or she is able to maintain a healthy balance of probiotics in his body, it can significantly reduce his or her potential risk of asthma attacks and anaphylactic shocks.

Sending Reinforcements: How to Promote Probiotic Growth

Now that you know the role of probiotics and how they overcome the harmful substances and pathogens that enter your body, the next big question is this, what can you do to help strengthen your gut's probiotic bacteria? How do you send "reinforcements," so to speak?

The answer is quite simple, and it is to eat foods rich in natural probiotics. Take note that children who were breastfed grow up with a stronger immune system compared to those who grew up on formula. This is because the mother's breastmilk is a natural source of probiotics. Formulas and processed milk, on the other hand, underwent a lot of processing that not only kills the harmful microbes in the milk but also the probiotics. Thus, breastfed children from the earliest point in their life already have a healthy balance of probiotics in their intestinal tract while those who are not are more susceptible to illness.

Fortunately, regardless of whether you were breastfed as a child or not, you can still adjust your lifestyle to support a healthy intestinal tract. By eating probiotic foods every day, for instance, you can get a good dose of probiotics.

Fermented vegetables are among the simplest yet most effective sources of probiotics. Fresh vegetables and fruits already contain microorganisms, especially if they are organically grown. These bacteria came from the plant sources' natural environment – soil, air, water, and so on. Some are harmful while others are beneficial and, as soon as the produce is harvested, the battle between these two general types of bacteria begins.

Left to fend for themselves, the probiotics in the vegetables and fruit will eventually diminish, leading to the development of harmful molds and yeasts starting with the damaged areas of the produce. The only way to help preserve the probiotics is to ferment them.

How exactly does fermentation help preserve the probiotics and nutrients in the vegetables and fruits? To answer this, let us first take a good look at the main ingredient for vegetable fermentation: salt. The role of salt is to draw the natural juices out of the cells of produce. When these juices combine with the salt, it becomes brine.

Lactobacillus acidophilus or lactic acid bacteria, the main probiotic, can survive in a briny environment because it does not need oxygen. Harmful bacteria, on the other hand, do and so they cannot survive in the brine.

Moreover, salt significantly reduces the likelihood of yeasts developing in the vegetable. Take note that yeasts are responsible for breaking down the fruit or vegetable's natural sugars to turn into alcohol instead of lactic acid. If you want to be exact in your measurements to promote lactic acid development instead of alcohol, then you need to make sure that the salinity of your brine is at 3.5 percent.

This is achievable if you have a 0.8 to 1.5 percent salt to vegetable weight ratio. It is important to have just the right amount of salt instead of having excessive amounts of it, though, because too much can also prevent lactic acid bacteria from flourishing.

Aside from providing you with probiotics, fermented vegetables will also make the natural vitamins and minerals in them become easier to digest. In fact, fermentation boosts the absorbability of vitamins and minerals naturally found in the vegetables, particularly the B vitamins and vitamin C. According to microbiologists, for instance, the iron in fermented vegetable juice is over 15 percent more absorbable by the body than fresh, raw vegetable juice.

So, have these facts increased your appetite for fermented vegetables? Hopefully, they have because they are so beneficial to your health. It is important to eat fermented vegetables every day not only because they have several health benefits but also because you can enjoy their flavor and texture. You can easily purchase fermented vegetables at a local grocery store but the best kind is always that which you make yourself because you are certain of their ingredients not to mention the fact that it is cheaper to make them yourself

However, before you start purchasing sea salt, cabbages, and whatnot, it is of utmost importance to create the ideal environment for fermentation. The next chapter will show you how to do just that.

Chapter 2 – Setting Up a Probiotic-Friendly Kitchen

Fermentation is a food preparation process that has been practiced for thousands of years, be it in five-star restaurants or the humble kitchens of a countryside home. This simply goes to show that you do not have to purchase any fancy and expensive equipment to start fermenting vegetables in your own kitchen.

All the same, there are important rules to follow and tools to prepare to ensure that your fermented vegetables turn out edible and beneficial. You certainly would not want to waste time, money, and effort into making them only to end up with a jar full of icky mold. This is why it is important for you to read this chapter first right before you start chopping and salting your vegetables.

In this chapter, you will learn about the five factors that affect the way your vegetables will ferment. You will also learn about the different equipment you need for fermenting vegetables. Moreover, if you have any doubts regarding your own skills and knowledge towards fermenting vegetables then this chapter will grant you the confidence in knowing that you are following the right steps.

The Five Factors that Affect Fermentation

The ideal environment for fermentation is dependent on five factors - light, temperature, pH level, time, and oxygen. We will go deeper into each of them so that you can control them as you re-create the wonderful fermented vegetable recipes found in the next chapter. Later on, you might even be able to make your own recipes based on your own and your family's personal preferences in terms of flavor, texture and overall appeal.

- **Light**

    Fermentation only transpires in a dark and cool environment. Direct sunlight is your enemy because it causes fluctuations in the temperature of your fermenting vegetables, leading to an imbalance in the development of probiotics.

    This does not mean, however, that you have to place your jar of pickling vegetables in a pitch-black shelf. Rather, place it in an area where there is no direct sunlight yet is also one where you can keep a good eye on it.

- **Temperature**

    The ideal temperature for fermentation is between the range of 55 and 75 degrees F, because it creates the perfect setting for lactobacilli to grow. It is important for the temperature to be consistent so that the fermentation process will remain undisrupted.

The lower the temperature is, the longer it takes for the fermentation process to occur. Thus, they may not be able to proliferate fast enough to protect the vegetable from rotting. On the other hand, the higher the temperature is, the faster it will occur, but if it is anything higher than the range given, it will not give the probiotics enough time to develop properly. The result will be ill-tasting fermented vegetables with underdeveloped acidity.

- **pH Level**

To refresh your memory on what pH level is exactly, it is the means of measuring the acidity or alkalinity of a solution using a scale from 0 to 14. A pH level of 7 is considered neutral, with anything beyond it considered as alkaline and anything below it as acidic.

Now, regarding fermentation, the exact pH level for vegetables to be considered as perfectly fermented is 4.6 and below. You can use a pH test strip to determine the acidity level of your vegetables as they ferment, but it is not necessary. Often, people simply taste test their fermented vegetables to determine if they are wonderfully sour enough to their liking.

- **Time**

The fermentation process takes a lot of time before you can move the fermented vegetables into the refrigerator to stall or significantly slow it down. Some vegetables take more time to ferment than others because it is all a matter of how long it takes to break down their starches based on the conditions of other factors.

It is also worth noting that the length of time given to the fermentation process can affect the type of probiotic species that will proliferate in the jar. However, unless you have the necessary tools to check, you cannot be certain as to which colonies thrive at that point in time.

Time also greatly affects the flavor and texture of the fermented vegetables. For instance, sauerkraut is typically given 3 to 9 days to ferment. The closer it is to the 9th day, the stronger the sourness is. Since fermented vegetables only deliver their health benefits when you actually enjoy eating them every day, it is ultimately up to your taste buds on how long you want to ferment them.

- **Oxygen**

The key to keeping lactobacilli alive in – and harmful bacteria and yeast away from – your fermented vegetables is through the oxygen-free brine. Any part of the vegetable that goes beyond the surface of the brine will immediately be festered with molds, yeasts, and aerobic bacteria, so it is important to check your fermenting vegetables periodically.

You can either add more brine, if necessary, or press down on the vegetables to ensure that they stay submerged. If there is any sign of scum, then you need to skim it off. However, it is important not to disturb the fermentation process by checking too often. Some people tend to open and close the jar too much, causing yeast spores and oxygen to enter the environment. This can lead the harmful bacteria to reduce the acidity level of the brine, thus promoting rot.

Always keep these five key factors in mind as you wait for your vegetables to ferment. Set the right environment for fermentation and you have a guarantee that you will get the flavors, textures, and probiotic benefits that you want.

Fermentation Equipment Tips and Tricks

Now that you know of the different factors that affect the fermentation of your vegetables, the next step is to prepare the right equipment. At the very least, all you need are the following: an extra sharp knife, a nice clean cutting board, a mixing bowl, a large mason jar, some salt, and of course, your vegetables.

In preparing your vegetables, the first thing you need to do is to chop them up. The smaller the pieces are, the faster they are likely to ferment, so keep that in mind. Aside from using a knife and cutting board, you can also use a food processor to slice, chop, or shred your vegetables.

Next, you need to have a bowl large enough to contain all your ingredients and, at the same time, allow you to toss and mix them without anything spilling over. Try to use a bowl made of non-reactive material, such as glassware, stoneware, wood, silicone, high quality stainless steel, or BPA-free hard plastic. As for the tools to use for tossing and mixing, perfectly clean hands are all you will ever need.

Now, once your vegetables are mixed and starting to sweat out the brine, you are going to need a sturdy vessel where you can store them as they ferment. It is important to avoid using a reactive material, as fermented foods are acidic. Therefore, you should try to avoid any vessel made with aluminum, cast iron, copper, low-quality stainless steel, and plastics containing BPA or bisphenol A, and/or PVC or polyvinyl chloride.

Opt for anything made with the same materials enumerated in the previous paragraph. Most people love to use either glass (mason) jars or crocks, so you can safely stick with those if you want to be sure. Here are some suggestions:

- **Glass Jars**

  It is no wonder that many people prefer to store their fermented vegetables in glass jars. They are cheap while also allowing you to see what is going on inside them. In addition, they come in many shapes and sizes so you can create a simple starter batch or half a year's worth of fermented vegetables with them.

The downside for most glass jars is that they tend to cause the brine to overflow because they do not add much weight to prevent the formation of air pockets during the fermentation process. In addition, most people need to wrap their glass jars in kitchen towels to minimize the penetration of light into the fermenting vegetables.

- **Ceramic Crocks**

Ceramic crocks are the traditional means of storing fermented vegetables and to this day, they are the perfect choice. Just make sure they do not contain lead. Take note that crocks can be quite heavy so if you are planning to make huge batches of fermented vegetables, you will need to keep this in mind.

- **Onggi Pots**

If you are a big fan of Korean food and you want to make your own kimchi, then know that the traditional vessel for storing it is the onggi pot. It is a clay pot made in such a way that it allows the fermentation gases to escape through its tiny pores. This leads to better flavor and texture of the kimchi.

Naturally, it is not too easy to find an onggi pot unless you live in Korea. However, if you do your homework, you can find a seasoned potter who knows how to make one for you.

- **Water-seal Crocks**

    If you want to take your vegetable fermentation hobby to the next level, then you might want to invest in water-seal crocks from Germany and Poland. These fancy but highly effective crocks have an air-lock feature, which allows the carbon dioxide to escape from it without letting oxygen into it.

After preparing a vessel where you can store your fermented vegetables, the next step is to find the right weight to place on top of them. It is important to put a kind of weight above your fermenting vegetables and brine, unless you are using a water-seal crock. This will minimize the possibility of the brine overflowing, because this is a natural result of the fermentation process. Specifically, the lactobacilli will start to produce a lot of carbon dioxide, which is what causes the brine to bubble over. The right weight can help keep this from happening.

Most people like to use the traditional clean smooth stone to keep the vegetables down. However, you will need to find a lime-free stone small enough to fit into the mouth of your vessel and large enough to hold down all your vegetables. You can also place a sheet of food-grade plastic wrap over your vegetables then add any kind of nonreactive weight over it. Some like to place a freezer bag on top of the fermenting vegetables then fill it up with water to act as a weight.

A nifty tool to have, especially if you are new to the world of fermenting vegetables, is the airlock. This tool is secured to the lid of the vessel – specifically a jar – to keep the outside air from entering the vessel yet allow the carbon dioxide to escape, thereby preventing the brine from overflowing. You can purchase jars with built-in airlocks at many home goods stores nowadays.

Finally, you will need a covering to shield your jar or crock of fermenting vegetables from the insects, pests, dust, and other contaminants in the outside world. At the same time, it should let the carbon dioxide escape from the vessel. The most commonly used covering is cheesecloth secured with rubber bands, but you can also use any clean cloth.

There you have it – all the tools you ever really need to start fermenting vegetables. Eventually, you might discover that you need more equipment later on but that is only when you have special preferences.

Now, here are just some sanitation steps to master before you start fermenting any vegetables or other probiotic foods at home:

Step 1: Clean and sanitize all equipment and work surfaces using hot water and eco-friendly soap.

Step 2: Use cool water to rinse the vegetables. You may mix in some vinegar into the water to remove any impurities from the surface of the vegetables, especially if they are not from an organic source.

Step 3: Sanitize the fermentation vessel by washing and scrubbing it thoroughly before rinsing and soaking in hot water.

Step 4: Once the vessel is filled with the vegetables and brine, place it on top of a tray to catch any brine that might overflow.

Step 5: Ensure that the fermentation occurs in an area with a constant temperature between 55 and 75 degrees F. This area is ideally not in the kitchen because the temperature tends to fluctuate in it.

Step 6: Never forget to transfer the fermented vegetables into the refrigerator as soon as they have reached the desired level of fermentation.

Lastly, if it looks slimy and gross and if it smells rotten, do yourself a favor by tossing it out and charging it to experience. You can definitely do better next time.

Chapter 3 – Choosing the Best Ingredients

Anyone can feel overwhelmed by the number of options one has upon entering a grocery store. You might even be surprised upon seeing the variety of salts you will encounter. There is no need to worry, though, for this chapter will show you some simple guidelines to help you choose the best ingredients for your fermentation project.

Salt

Sea salt is the quintessential ingredient in fermentation, with kosher pickling salt as its close second. However, feel free to use a variety of salts, provided you inquire of the change in measurements. Some salts are particularly stronger than others, so avoid relying on the same measurements for sea salt if you want to use, say, gray salt. Also, avoid salts with additives.

The best salts for fermentation are:

- Kosher pickling salt

- Sea salt

- Himalayan crystal salt

- Gray salt, or *sel gris*

- Flower of salt, or *fleur de sel*

Avoid iodized salt whenever possible, for iodine has antimicrobial properties that can prevent the development of the probiotics. Also, avoid industrialized refined salt due to the possible unnecessary additives in them.

Greens and Brassicas

Greens and brassicas such as cabbage, napa cabbage, and spinach are among the most commonly used ingredients in making fermented vegetables. When shopping for them, make sure to inspect the leaves closely. There should be little to no limp and wilted leaves, and they should be springy when you touch them.

Roots, Shoots, and Tubers

Root and tuber vegetables such as radishes, carrots, and jicama are quite easy to pickle and add to relishes and krauts. Make sure to pick the ones that are well-formed and firm. Avoid anything with green patches or with sprouts.

When it comes to shoots, choose those with firm stalks that are roughly of the same thickness. This will ensure that the shoots will all ferment together in generally the same time.

Mushrooms

When it comes to choosing mushrooms for pickling, make sure to find the ones with a fresh, earthy smell. They should also be nice, firm, and with minimal to no blemishes.

Nightshades

Nightshades such as eggplants, peppers, and tomatoes should feel heavy, with flesh that bounce back if you gently press against it. Also, pick those with the smoothest and shiniest skin to get the best quality for fermenting.

Cucumbers

Pickling cucumbers have relatively thicker skin than those used in salads and other dishes. Choose the ones that are evenly green with no patches of yellow to ensure their crispness even as they go through the fermentation process.

With all these in mind, choose vegetables as well as fruits that are newly picked, in-season, and locally produced. Perhaps it is best to choose the recipes to start with based on what is in season. That way, you have a guarantee regarding their freshness, flavor, texture, and overall quality.

Chapter 4 – Fermented Vegetable Recipes

Classic Sauerkraut

Yields: 1 ½ quarts

You will need:

- 3 lbs. green and/or red cabbage
- 1 ½ Tbsp sea salt

How to Prepare:

Rinse the cabbage and discard any withered or bruised outer leaves. Slice in half across the core. Then, slice into thin strips with a sharp knife. Alternatively, slice the cabbage halves into larger chunks and shred in the food processor.

Place the shredded cabbage into a large bowl and sprinkle in the salt. Massage the salt into the cabbage until the liquids start to get drawn out of the leaves. Continue to massage and squeeze to draw out as much water as possible.

Stuff the shredded cabbage into a clean jar along with the liquids. Press down on the cabbage to make sure that the leaves are completely submerged in the liquids. There should be an inch of space between the rim and the mixture. Cover the jar with a cheesecloth secured with rubber bands.

Place the sauerkraut in a cool shelf away from direct sunlight, with a temperature approximately between 50 and 75 degrees F.

Allow the sauerkraut to ferment from three to nine days, checking once every other day by checking the smell and taste. Always pack down firmly on the shredded cabbage to keep them completely submerged.

Once you are satisfied with the flavor of the sauerkraut, transfer the jar into the refrigerator and refrigerate for up to 6 months.

BLAUKRAUT

Yields: 2 quarts

You will need:

- 3 lbs. red cabbage
- 1 small onion
- 2 crisp tart apples
- 1 Tbsp caraway seeds
- 1 Tbsp sea salt

How to Prepare:

Rinse the cabbage and discard any withered or bruised outer leaves. Slice in half across the core then slice into thin strips with a sharp knife. Alternatively, slice the cabbage halves into larger chunks and shred in the food processor.

Place the shredded cabbage into a large bowl. Thinly slice the onion and add into the bowl. Remove the core from each apple then quarter and slice thinly. Add the sliced apple into the bowl.

Sprinkle the caraway seeds into the bowl of cabbage then add the salt. Massage everything well with clean hands, adding more salt if needed.

Massage the salt into the cabbage until the liquids start to get drawn out of the leaves. Continue to massage and squeeze to draw out as much water as possible.

Stuff the shredded cabbage, apple, and onion mixture into a clean jar along with the liquids. Press down on the cabbage to make sure that the leaves are completely submerged in the liquids. There should be an inch of space between the rim and the mixture. Cover the jar with a cheesecloth secured with rubber bands.

Place the blaukraut in a cool shelf away from direct sunlight, with a temperature approximately between 50 and 75 degrees F.

Allow the blaukraut to ferment from 7 to 14 days. Each day, make sure that the shredded cabbage is completely submerged in the brine. After the 7th day, begin checking the kraut every day by testing the smell and taste.

Once you are satisfied with the flavor of the blaukraut, transfer the jar into the refrigerator and refrigerate for up to 12 months.

Gingered Carrot Kraut

Yields: 2 quarts

You will need:

- 4 lbs. carrots
- ½ lemon
- 1 Tbsp. freshly grated ginger
- 1 Tbsp. sea salt

How to Prepare:

Peel and grate the carrots into a large bowl. Add the freshly grated ginger then juice and zest the lemon over the mixture.

Stir in the salt and massage everything until the liquids start to come out. Continue to massage and squeeze to draw out as much water as possible.

Stuff the gingered carrot mixture into a clean jar along with the liquids. Press down on the carrot mixture to make sure that it is completely submerged in the liquids. You can use a sheet of food-grade plastic wrap or other type of weight to keep the carrots submerged.

There should be an inch of space between the rim and the mixture. Cover the jar with a cheesecloth secured with rubber bands.

Place the blaukraut in a cool shelf away from direct sunlight, with a temperature approximately between 50 and 75 degrees F.

Allow the blaukraut to ferment from 7 to 14 days. Each day, make sure that the shredded cabbage is completely submerged in the brine. After the 7th day, begin checking the kraut every day by testing the smell and taste.

Once you are satisfied with the flavor of the gingered carrot kraut, transfer the jar into the refrigerator and refrigerate for up to 12 months.

Celeriac Kraut

Yields: ½ quart

You will need:

- 1 lb. celeriac root

- ¾ tsp. sea salt

How to Prepare:

Scrub the celeriac root clean and then peel and shred using a sharp knife or grater. Place inside a large bowl and sprinkle in the salt. Massage the salt into the shredded celeriac until the liquids are drawn out. Continue to massage and squeeze to draw out as much water as possible.

Stuff the shredded celeriac into a clean jar along with the liquids. Press down on the celeriac to make sure that it is completely submerged in the liquids. There should be an inch of space between the rim and the mixture. Cover the jar with a cheesecloth secured with rubber bands.

Place the celeriac kraut in a cool shelf away from direct sunlight, with a temperature approximately between 50 and 75 degrees F.

Allow the celeriac kraut to ferment from five to ten days. Always pack down firmly on the shredded celeriac kraut to keep them completely submerged. After the 5th day, start taste testing the kraut to determine how sour you want it.

Once you are satisfied with the flavor of the celeriac kraut, transfer the jar into the refrigerator and refrigerate for up to 6 months.

Cauliflower Kraut

Yields: 1 ½ quarts

You will need:

- 2 lbs. cauliflower
- 3 jalapeno peppers
- 2 ½ tsp. sea salt

How to Prepare:

Rinse the cauliflower in cold running water then quarter and slice into thin pieces. Place in a bowl and set aside.

Chop the jalapeno peppers and discard the seeds. Add to the cauliflower with the salt and toss several times to coat. Cover the bowl with a kitchen towel and set aside for 30 minutes.

After 30 minutes, toss the cauliflower again several times before transferring into a clean jar. If the cauliflower does not look like there is enough brine, it is fine. Place a weight above it, such as a plastic bag filled with water, before sealing to press down on the cauliflower and allow it to shed its liquids. Give it 8 hours.

After 8 hours, press the cauliflower down into the brine until it is completely submerged. You can repeat the bag trick if there still is not enough brine, although in most cases, it is not necessary.

Once the cauliflower is sufficiently submerged in its brine, cover the jar with a cheesecloth secured with rubber bands and set aside to ferment for 4 to 8 days in a cool, dry place.

Each day, check to ensure that the cauliflower stays submerged. Taste test after the 4th day until the cauliflower kraut is sour enough to your liking. Once it is, seal with the lid and refrigerate. Consume within 9 months.

Zesty Lemon Kraut

Yields: 1 ½ quarts

You will need:

- 3 lbs. green cabbage
- ¾ cups julienned fresh mint leaves
- 1 ½ lemons
- 1 ½ Tbsp sea salt

How to Prepare:

Rinse the cabbage and discard any withered or bruised outer leaves. Slice in half across the core. Then slice into thin strips with a sharp knife. Alternatively, slice the cabbage halves into larger chunks and shred in the food processor.

Place the shredded cabbage into a large bowl and sprinkle in the salt. Massage the salt into the cabbage until the liquids start to get drawn out of the leaves. Continue to massage and squeeze to draw out as much water as possible. Set aside.

Juice and zest the lemon then add it to the cabbage mixture along with the mint. Mix everything well with clean hands.

Stuff the shredded cabbage mixture into a clean jar along with the liquids. Press down on the cabbage to submerge the leaves completely in the liquids. There should be an inch of space between the rim and the mixture. Cover the jar with a cheesecloth secured with rubber bands.

Place the sauerkraut in a cool shelf away from direct sunlight, with a temperature approximately between 50 and 75 degrees F.

Allow the sauerkraut to ferment from three to nine days, checking once every other day by checking the smell and taste. Always pack down firmly on the shredded cabbage to keep them completely submerged.

Once you are satisfied with the flavor of the sauerkraut, transfer the jar into the refrigerator and refrigerate for up to 6 months.

Zesty Spinach Kraut

Yields: 1 ½ quarts

You will need:

- 3 lb. chopped spinach leaves
- 2 medium sweet onions
- 3 Tbsp. freshly ground lemon juice
- 1 ¾ Tbsp. crumbled dried oregano
- 3 tsp. sea salt

How to Prepare:

Peel the sweet onions then slice them into quarters before slicing them thinly. Place the chopped sweet onions into the bowl and add the salt. Mix well then cover the bowl with a kitchen cloth. Set aside for 30 minutes to sweat.

After 30 minutes, uncover the bowl of onions and stir in the lemon juice, oregano, and spinach. Mix well gently, taking care not to bruise the spinach leaves. Add more salt, if necessary.

Place the mixture into a clean jar, pressing down on the mixture to ensure that everything is submerged in the liquids. There should be an inch of space between the rim and the mixture. Cover the jar with a cheesecloth secured with rubber bands.

Place the spinach kraut in a cool shelf away from direct sunlight, with a temperature approximately between 50 and 75 degrees F.

Allow the spinach kraut to ferment from four to ten days. Always ensure that solids are completely submerged in the brine.

After day 4, begin taste testing the kraut. Once you are satisfied with the flavor, cover the jar with its lid and transfer into the refrigerator. Serve within 6 months.

Curtido Rojo

Yields: 2 quarts

You will need:

- ½ red or green cabbage
- ¼ lb green beans
- 1 beet
- 1 small red onion
- 1 large garlic clove
- 1 bay leaf
- ½ to 1 fresh jalapeno pepper
- 1 Tbsp. sea salt
- ½ Tbsp. crumbled dried oregano
- ½ Tbsp. cumin seeds
- ½ Tbsp. freshly grated lime or orange zest

How to Prepare:

Rinse the cabbage and discard any withered or bruised outer leaves. Slice in half across the core. Then slice into thin strips with a sharp knife. Alternatively, slice the cabbage halves into larger chunks and shred in the food processor.

Place the shredded cabbage into a large bowl and sprinkle in the salt.

Peel the beet and rinse thoroughly in running water. Shred with a box grater or food processor and add into the bowl of cabbage.

Massage the salt into the cabbage and beets until the liquids start to be drawn out. Continue to massage and squeeze to draw out as much water as possible. If the liquids are not enough, cover the bowl loosely with a kitchen towel and set aside for 30 minutes before squeezing again.

Peel the garlic and onions and slice thinly. Trim the green beans then slice into small pieces.

Add the garlic, onions, and green beans into the cabbage and beet mixture, followed by the zest, cumin seeds, red chili flakes, and oregano. Slice and seed the jalapeno pepper and mix in as well.

Once the mixture is ready, place the bay leaf into a large clean mason jar and add the mixture in. Ensure that the solids are completely submerged in the liquid and there is an inch of headspace between the rim and the liquid.

Cover the jar with a cheesecloth and secure it with rubber bands. Set on a cool, dry shelf away from direct sunlight from four to fourteen days. Ensure each day that the solids stay completely submerged. Skim off and discard any foam that forms on the surface.

Once the curtido rojo is pleasantly sour, cover and refrigerate. Consume within 6 months.

Basic Pickled Cucumbers

Yields: 2 lbs.

You will need:

- 2 lbs. small pickling cucumbers
- 2 cups non-chlorinated water
- 2 cups apple cider vinegar or red wine vinegar
- ¼ cup sea salt
- ½ cup sauerkraut juice

How to Prepare:

Place the cucumbers in a bowl of ice water and set aside for 30 minutes. Meanwhile, combine the sea salt, sauerkraut juice, vinegar, and non-chlorinated water in a clean pitcher and set aside.

Once chilled, slice the ends of the cucumbers and place them in a clean jar. Add the brine mixture and cover with a cheesecloth secured with rubber bands.

Place the jar of cucumbers on a cool, dry shelf away from direct sunlight. Allow to ferment between 3 to 9 days. Make sure to taste the cucumbers every two days. Skim off and discard any mold that grows over the brine. On the other hand, if the mold starts to grow roots, discard the mixture immediately.

Once the flavor is sour but the texture is still crunchy, transfer the pickles into the refrigerator and store. Serve within 6 months.

Pickled Asparagus

Yields: 1 ½ quarts

You will need:

- 2 ½ lbs asparagus spears
- 6 garlic cloves
- 3 to 6 dried red chilies
- 1 ½ bay leaves
- 6 cups non-chlorinated water
- 4 Tbsp sea salt
- 1 ½ tsp black peppercorns
- ¾ tsp chili pepper flakes

How to Prepare:

Stir the sea salt into the water until thoroughly dissolved. Set aside.

Crush and peel the garlic cloves then slice them into wedges. Set aside.

Spread the bay leaves, chili pepper flakes, and peppercorns inside a clean jar.

Trim off the tough ends of the asparagus spears then line them up in standing position inside the jar. Stuff the slivers of garlic in between. Ensure that the asparagus spears are tightly packed inside the jar.

Pour the brine over the asparagus, ensuring they are completely submerged. Leave about an inch of space between the rim of the jar and the brine. Cover the jar with a cheesecloth secured with rubber bands.

Place the jar in a cool, dry shelf for 5 to 8 days. Ensure that the asparagus stays completely submerged throughout the fermentation process.

Once the asparagus turns dark green, you are ready to transfer it to the refrigerator. Seal and refrigerate. Consume within 12 months.

Napa Cabbage Kimchi

Yields: 1 ½ quarts

You will need:

- 2 ½ lbs. napa cabbage
- ½ lb. daikon
- ¾ garlic bulb
- 2 medium onions
- 1 inch fresh gingerroot
- 3 cups non-chlorinated water
- ¾ cup Korean red pepper powder
- ½ cup sea salt
- ¼ cup chopped scallions
- 1 ½ Tbsp brown sugar or other sweetener
- 1 ½ tsp fish sauce

How to Prepare:

Combine the non-chlorinated water and salt in a pitcher and set aside.

Rinse the Napa cabbage then blot dry with paper towels. Place in a large, deep mixing bowl and set aside.

Peel the daikon radish and then slice thinly into diagonal strips. Add the daikon radish into the mixing bowl with the napa cabbage.

Pour the brine over the vegetables and turn several times to ensure they are coated. Cover with a kitchen towel and set aside in room temperature for 6 hours.

After 6 hours, drain thoroughly and place the vegetables in a colander. Rinse in non-chlorinated water and set aside to drain further.

In the meantime, separate the garlic cloves and crush them with the back of your knife to peel off the skins easily. Peel the onions as well as the ginger.

Place the garlic, onion, and ginger in a food processor and process until pasty, adding some non-chlorinated water, if needed. Alternatively, crush into a paste with a mortar and pestle.

Add the fish sauce, sweetener, and Korean red pepper into the food processor and blend well until smooth, adding more water, if needed.

Transfer the mixture into a large mixing bowl and add the chopped scallions. Using clean hands, massage the mixture onto the napa cabbage and daikon, making sure that all surfaces are completely covered. Season with more salt, if needed.

Transfer the kimchi into clean mason jars, pressing down on the solids to ensure that they are submerged in the brine. Cover with a cheesecloth secured with rubber bands, ensuring that there is at least 1 inch of space between the rim and the kimchi.

Set on a cool, dry shelf at room temperature for 3 to 9 days. Taste the kimchi once every two days. Once you are satisfied with the flavor and texture, transfer into the refrigerator to store. Serve within 6 months.

Arugula Kimchi

Yields: 1 quart

You will need:

- 21 oz. arugula
- 1/3 inch fresh ginger
- 6 garlic cloves
- 2 to 3 dried red chilies
- 2 cups non-chlorinated water
- 2 Tbsp brown sugar or other sweetener
- 2 tsp sea salt

How to Prepare:

In a glass pitcher, pour in the water, salt, and sugar. Stir well until the salt and sugar are dissolved then set aside.

Loosely roll up the arugula leaves and place them in a clean jar. Add the dried red chilies. Peel and grate the ginger into the jar. Crush and peel the garlic cloves and then slice and place inside the jar as well.

Pour the liquid mixture over the vegetables. Ensure that the leaves are completely submerged in the water, and that there is at least one inch of space between the rim of the jar and the liquid.

Cover the jar with a cheesecloth secured with rubber bands and place in a cool, dry place away from direct sunlight. Let it ferment for up to 5 days; ensure that the arugula stays completely submerged.

After two days, begin taste testing the kimchi. Once it is sour to your liking, cover with the lid and transfer into the refrigerator. Consume within 6 months.

Southern Fermented Coleslaw

Yields: 1 ½ quarts

You will need:

- 1 ½ lbs. green cabbage
- 1/3 lb celery root, or 1 ½ tsp celery seeds
- 1 large green bell pepper
- 1 large onion
- 1 large carrot
- 1 small apple
- ½ inch fresh ginger, peeled and grated
- ¼ cup coconut oil
- ¼ cup olive or sesame oil
- ¼ cup honey
- 2 Tbsp. sea salt, plus more, if needed
- 3 tsp dry mustard
- Freshly ground black pepper, to taste

How to Prepare:

Slice the cabbage into thin strips and place in a large bowl.

Slice the bell pepper in half, discard the core and stem, and slice into thin strips. Add to the bowl of cabbage.

Peel the onion and slice thinly. Place into the bowl as well.

With a box grater, grate the carrot, apple, and celery root and mix well into the bowl of vegetables.

Salt the vegetables and massage well with clean hands, squeezing until the liquids come out. Transfer the vegetables and liquids into a clean glass jar, ensuring that the vegetables are submerged in the liquids.

Cover the jar with a cheesecloth secured with rubber bands and place in a cool, dry shelf to ferment for 3 to 7 days. Taste the fermented vegetables once every two days and make sure that the solids remain submerged.

After about 7 days, drain the coleslaw thoroughly using a strainer, using a bowl to catch the liquids. Press out as much of the liquid as possible using a spoon. Place the fermented vegetables into a bowl.

Stir the honey, oils, and dry mustard into the liquids. Peel the ginger and grate over the mixture. Stir well to combine.

Pour the dressing over the fermented vegetables and mix well. Season to taste with salt and black pepper. Cover and refrigerate for up to 3 weeks.

SPICY BRUSSELS SPROUTS PICKLES

Yields: 1 ½ quarts

You will need:

- 1 ½ lbs. Brussels sprouts
- 7 garlic cloves
- 4 cups non-chlorinated water
- 3 Tbsp. smoked salt
- 3 Tbsp sea salt
- 1 ½ Tbsp. chili pepper flakes
- 1 ½ Tbsp. peppercorns
- 3 to 4 jalapeno peppers

How to Prepare:

Combine the water, smoked salt, and sea salt in a large pitcher. Stir until the salts are completely dissolved. Set aside.

Crush and peel the garlic cloves then scatter them in a large clean jar. Add the chili pepper flakes and peppercorns.

Seed and slice the jalapeno peppers. Slice the Brussels sprouts in half and place them in the jar al0ng with the jalapeno peppers.

Pour the brine over the mixture, ensuring that all the solids are completely submerged. Cover the jar with a cheesecloth secured with rubber bands and place in a cool, dry place away from direct sunlight. Let it ferment for 7 to 14 days. Make sure that the vegetables stay completely submerged.

After a week, start taste testing the Brussels sprouts. When they are sour enough to your liking, cover with the lid and transfer into the refrigerator. Consume within 6 months.

Pickled Carrot Sticks

Yields: 1 quart

You will need:

- 2 lbs. carrots

- 4 cups non-chlorinated water

- ¼ cup sea salt

- 1 Tbsp brown sugar or other sweetener

How to Prepare:

Stir the sea salt and sugar into the water until thoroughly dissolved. Set aside.

Peel the carrots and then slice them into sticks, about ¼ inches in width and 3 to 4 inches in length, or as desired.

Place the carrot sticks into a clean jar and add enough brine to cover them completely. You may use a sheet of food-grade plastic wrap or other type of weight to keep them submerged.

Cover the jar with a cheesecloth secured with rubber bands and place in a cool, dry place away from direct sunlight. Let it ferment for 7 to 14 days. Ensure that the carrots stay completely submerged. If any mold starts to form on top, remove and discard right away.

After a week, start taste testing the pickled carrot sticks. When they are sour enough to your liking, cover with the lid and transfer into the refrigerator. Consume within 12 months.

Vietnamese Daikon and Carrot Pickles

Yields: 1 quart

You will need:

- 1 lb. carrots
- 1 lb. daikon radishes
- 4 cups non-chlorinated water
- ¼ cup sea salt
- 1 Tbsp brown sugar or other sweetener

How to Prepare:

Stir the sea salt and sugar into the water until thoroughly dissolved. Set aside.

Peel the carrots and radishes, and then julienne them using a sharp knife or food processor. Place them into a large clean jar and add enough brine to cover them fully. You may use a sheet of food-grade plastic wrap or other type of weight to keep them submerged.

Cover the jar with a cheesecloth secured with rubber bands and place in a cool, dry place away from direct sunlight. Do the fermentation process for 7 to 14 days; ensure that the vegetables stay completely submerged. If any mold starts to form on top, remove and discard right away.

After a week, start taste testing the carrot and daikon radish pickles. When they are sour enough to your liking, cover with the lid and transfer into the refrigerator. Consume within 12 months.

Japanese Pickled Cabbage

Yields: 1 ½ quarts

You will need:

- 2 ½ lbs. napa cabbage

- 1 ½ Tbsp. sea salt

How to Prepare:

Rinse the napa cabbage and then blot dry with paper towels. Chop into half-inch pieces and place in a large, deep mixing bowl.

Sprinkle the napa cabbage with salt and massage all over until the liquid starts to come out. Cover the bowl with the kitchen towel and set aside for 45 minutes to an hour to let the napa cabbage continue to sweat.

After letting it stand, transfer the napa cabbage and liquids into a clean jar. Make sure the cabbage is completely submerged in the brine.

Cover the jar with a cheesecloth secured with rubber bands and place in a cool, dry place away from direct sunlight. Ferment for 7 to 14 days; ensure that the napa cabbage stays completely submerged.

After a week, start taste testing the cabbage. When it is sour enough based on your own preferences, cover with the lid and transfer into the refrigerator. Consume within 8 months.

Coriander Pickles

Yields: ½ quart

You will need:

- 2 cups non-chlorinated water

- ½ cup green coriander seeds

- 4 tsp. sea salt

How to Prepare:

Stir the sea salt into the water until thoroughly dissolved. Set aside.

Pour the green coriander seeds into a small clean jar then add just enough brine to keep the seeds completely submerged. Line the surface with food-grade plastic wrap, if desired, to prevent the seeds from rising above the brine.

Cover the jar with a cheesecloth secured with rubber bands and place in a cool, dry place away from direct sunlight. Ferment for 4 to 7 days; ensure that the seeds stay completely submerged. If any mold starts to form on top, remove and discard right away.

When the seeds are sour enough to your liking, cover with the lid and transfer into the refrigerator. Consume within 6 months.

Spiced Cherry Tomato Pickles

Yields: 2 quarts

You will need:

- 2 ½ lbs. cherry tomatoes
- 2 quarts non-chlorinated water
- ½ head garlic
- 1/3 cup sea salt
- ½ tsp. mustard seeds
- ½ tsp. coriander seeds
- ½ tsp. peppercorns
- 2 Tbsp. chopped fresh basil leaves
- 2 Tbsp. chopped fresh flat leaf parsley
- Chili pepper flakes, to taste

How to Prepare:

Crush and peel the garlic, and then slice into slivers. Set aside.

Combine the water and sea salt in a pitcher. Stir until the salt is completely dissolved. Set aside.

Rinse the tomatoes thoroughly and then place them in a large clean jar. Stuff in the basil, parsley, garlic slivers, peppercorns, and mustard and coriander seeds in between the spaces of the tomatoes. Sprinkle in the chili pepper flakes.

Pour the brine into the mixture until everything is completely submerged. Cover the jar with a cheesecloth secured with rubber bands and place in a cool, dry place away from direct sunlight.

Ferment for 6 to 8 days; ensure that the mixture stays completely submerged. If any mold starts to form on top, remove and discard right away.

After day 6, you can start taste tasting the spiced cherry tomato pickles. When they are sour enough to your liking and tender, cover the jar with the lid and transfer into the refrigerator.

Let the tomatoes stand in the refrigerator for 7 to 14 days before serving. Consume within 6 months.

Shiitake Mushroom Pickles

Yields: 1 ½ quarts

You will need:

- 4 ½ cups dried shiitake mushrooms
- 1 ½ quarts non-chlorinated water
- 5 garlic cloves
- 4 whole dried chilies
- 1 ½ bay leaves
- 1 ½ Tbsp. sea salt
- 1 ½ tsp. peppercorns

How to Prepare:

Place the dried mushrooms into a bowl and add the water. Cover the bowl with a kitchen towel and set aside for 3 hours to let the mushrooms rehydrate.

After 3 hours, strain the mushrooms, reserving the soaking liquid in a bowl. Filter the liquid with a coffee filter or cheesecloth-lined strainer to remove the grit. Then, add the salt to the liquid and stir well. Set aside.

Rinse the mushrooms thoroughly and discard the woody stems, then set aside.

Crush and peel the garlic cloves. Place half the cloves into a clean jar. Add half the red chilies, followed by peppercorns and mushrooms. Repeat with the second layer. Add the brine, ensuring that everything is thoroughly submerged.

Place a plastic bag into the jar over the mixture and fill it with water to add pressure to the mixture and keep it packed. Cover the jar with a cheesecloth secured with rubber bands and place in a cool, dry place away from direct sunlight.

Ferment for 7 to 10 days; ensure that the garlic paste stays completely submerged. After day 7, start taste testing the shiitake mushroom pickles. When they are sour enough to your liking, cover with the lid, transfer to the refrigerator, and consume within 2 months.

SPICY MEXICAN-STYLE PICKLES

Yields: 2 quarts

You will need:

- 1 lb. chopped cauliflower
- 1 lb. carrots
- 1 lb. jalapeno peppers, or ¾ Tbsp. chili pepper flakes
- 1 small onion
- 3 garlic cloves
- 8 cups non-chlorinated water
- 4 Tbsp. sea salt
- 1 Tbsp. crumbled dried oregano

How to Prepare:

Mix the water and sea salt in a pitcher until the salt dissolves completely. Set aside.

Slice the onion into wedges. Remove the core off the jalapeno peppers. Peel and slice the carrots, onions, and garlic. Place everything into a large bowl.

Add the cauliflower into the bowl of vegetables along with the dried oregano. Mix everything well before transferring into a large clean jar. Pour in the brine until the mixture is completely submerged. You can use a sheet of food-grade plastic wrap or other type of weight to keep the solids submerged.

Cover the jar with a cheesecloth secured with rubber bands and place in a cool, dry place away from direct sunlight. Ferment for 7 to 21 days; ensure that the vegetables stay completely submerged. If you notice the vegetables losing their color, do not worry for that is normal.

After a week, start taste testing the vegetables. When it is sour enough to your liking, you can transfer them into small jars then cover with the lid. Store in the refrigerator and consume within 12 months.

Celery Relish

Yields: ½ quart

You will need:

- ¾ lb. celery stalk and leaves
- 5 fresh sage leaves
- ½ Tbsp. chopped fresh thyme
- ½ tsp sea salt

How to Prepare:

Finely chop the celery stalk and leaves as well as the sage leaves. Place inside a bowl along with the chopped fresh thyme. Add the sea salt and massage everything well until they start to sweat. Cover the bowl with a kitchen towel and set aside for half an hour.

Once the celery has released a good amount of brine, transfer everything into a clean jar. Press down on the celery mixture to ensure it is submerged in the brine. You can use a sheet of food-grade plastic wrap or other type of weight to keep the solids submerged.

Cover the jar with a cheesecloth secured with rubber bands and place in a cool, dry place away from direct sunlight. Ferment for

5 to 10 days; ensure that the vegetables stay completely submerged.

After 5 days, start taste testing the celery relish. When it is sour enough to your liking, you can transfer them into small jars and then cover with the lid. Store in the refrigerator and consume within 10 months.

Fermented Cilantro

Yields: ½ quart

You will need:

- 1 lb. cilantro

- 1 tsp. sea salt

How to Prepare:

Slice the stems off the cilantro leaves and place the leaves in a bowl. Add the salt and toss to coat. Cover the bowl with a kitchen towel and set aside for 30 minutes to give them time to sweat.

After 30 minutes, continue to massage the leaves and then transfer into a clean jar. Ensure that the leaves are completely submerged in the brine. You can use a sheet of food-grade plastic wrap or other type of weight to keep the solids submerged.

Cover the jar with a cheesecloth secured with rubber bands and place in a cool, dry place away from direct sunlight. Let it ferment for 4 to 7 days; ensure that the leaves stay completely submerged.

After day 4, start taste testing the vegetables. When it is sour enough to your liking, you can transfer them into small jars and then cover with the lid. Store in the refrigerator and consume within 6 months.

Spiced Collard Green Relish

Yields: 1 ½ quarts

You will need:

- 2 ½ lbs. collard greens
- 8 garlic cloves
- 2 small onions
- 3 jalapeno peppers
- 4 ½ Tbsp freshly grated ginger
- 2 ½ tsp. sea salt
- 1 to 1 ½ tsp. ground cardamom

How to Prepare:

Rinse and drain the collard greens, and then chop off the stems. Roll the leaves up together, and then slice thinly. Place into a large bowl and some of the salt. Massage the collard greens until they start to sweat. Add more salt, if needed.

Mince the garlic, jalapeno peppers and onion then add into the bowl of collard greens. Stir in the cardamom and ginger and then mix well.

Stuff the mixture into a clean jar, making sure that the vegetables are completely submerged in the brine. You can use a sheet of food-grade plastic wrap or other type of weight to keep the mixture submerged.

Cover the jar with a cheesecloth secured with rubber bands and place in a cool, dry place away from direct sunlight. Ferment for 5 to 10 days; ensure that the mixture stays completely submerged.

After day 5, start taste testing the collard green relish. When it is sour enough to your liking, you can transfer them into small jars and then cover with the lid. Store in the refrigerator and consume within 6 months.

Sweet Corn Relish

Yields: 1 ½ quarts

You will need:

- 4 ½ cups raw sweet corn kernels
- 1 small zucchini
- 1 large red onion
- 1 large red bell pepper
- 4 ½ Tbsp. chopped cilantro
- 1 ½ Tbsp. raw honey
- 2 ½ tsp. sea salt

How to Prepare:

Core, seed, and dice the bell pepper. Dice the zucchini and red onion as well and then place everything into a large bowl. Add the corn kernels and cilantro. Season with the salt and mix everything well until the brine starts to form.

Once there is enough brine to cover the mixture, transfer everything into a clean jar. You can use a sheet of food-grade plastic wrap or other type of weight to keep the mixture submerged.

Cover the jar with a cheesecloth secured with rubber bands and place in a cool, dry place away from direct sunlight. Let it ferment for 3 to 4 days; ensure that the mixture stays completely submerged.

After day 3, start taste testing the sweet corn relish. When it has the perfect balance of sweet and sourness, stir in the honey and cover with the lid. Store in the refrigerator and consume within 1 month.

Fermented Eggplant

Yields: 1 ½ quarts

You will need:

- 2 ¼ lbs. eggplant
- 1 ¼ Tbsp. sea salt
- 2 garlic cloves
- 2 fresh basil leaves

How to Prepare:

Peel the eggplants and then slice into small cubes. Place the eggplant cubes into a bowl and sprinkle in the salt. Toss well to coat. Cover the bowl with a kitchen towel and set aside to allow the eggplant to sweat.

Once the eggplant has released sufficient brine, add the garlic and mix well. Transfer everything into a clean jar, ensuring that the mixture is completely submerged in the brine.

You can use a sheet of food-grade plastic wrap or other type of weight to keep the mixture submerged.

Cover the jar with a cheesecloth secured with rubber bands and place in a cool, dry place away from direct sunlight. Allow to ferment for 4 to 14 days; ensure that the mixture stays completely submerged.

After day 4, start taste testing the fermented eggplant. When it is sour enough to your liking, cover with the lid, transfer to the refrigerator, and consume within 10 months.

Garlic Paste

Yields: 1 cup

You will need:

- 4 garlic heads
- 1 tsp. sea salt

How to Prepare:

Separate the garlic cloves and crush each with the handle of a knife. Remove the skins and place the cloves into a food processor. Blend until pasty, then add the salt and blend again until combined.

Transfer the garlic paste into a clean jar. Place a plastic bag into the jar over the garlic paste and fill it with water to add pressure to the paste and keep it packed. Cover the jar with a cheesecloth secured with rubber bands and place in a cool, dry place away from direct sunlight. Allow to ferment for 14 to 21 days; ensure that the garlic paste stays completely submerged.

After day 14, start taste testing the garlic paste. When it is sour enough to your liking, cover with the lid, transfer to the refrigerator, and consume within 12 months.

Prepared Horseradish

Yields: 2 cups

You will need:

- 1 lb. horseradish root
- 1/3 cup freshly squeezed lemon juice
- 2 tsp. sea salt

How to Prepare:

Peel the horseradish root then slice into cubes. Place in a food processor and process into a paste. Add the salt and lemon juice and process again to combine.

Transfer the horseradish paste into a clean jar. Place a plastic bag into the jar over the horseradish paste and fill it with water to add pressure to the paste and keep it packed.

Cover the jar with a cheesecloth secured with rubber bands and place in a cool, dry place away from direct sunlight. Let it ferment for 3 to 7 days; ensure that the horseradish paste stays completely submerged.

After day 3, start taste testing the prepared horseradish. When it is sour enough to your liking, cover with the lid, transfer to the refrigerator, and consume within 12 months.

Onion Relish

Yields: 1 quart

You will need:

- 3 medium onions
- ¾ Tbsp. sea salt
- ½ Tbsp. ground cumin
- ½ Tbsp. mustard seeds
- ½ Tbsp. sauerkraut brine

How to Prepare:

Using a sharp knife, cut off the top and bottom ends of each onion. Then, remove the skins and any bruised areas. Slice the onions sharply into thin rings and place in a bowl.

Add the sea salt and toss well to coat then sprinkle in the cumin and mustard seeds. Toss well and then mix in the sauerkraut brine.

Transfer everything into a clean jar. Press down on the mixture to ensure that it is fully submerged in the brine. Place a plastic bag into the jar over the onion relish and fill it with water to add pressure to the relish and keep it packed.

Cover the jar with a cheesecloth secured with rubber bands and place in a cool, dry place away from direct sunlight. Ferment for 7 to 14 days; ensure that the onion relish stays completely submerged.

After day 7, start taste testing the onion relish. When it is sour enough to your liking, cover with the lid, transfer to the refrigerator, and consume within 18 months.

Chapter 5 – Other Probiotic Food Recipes

CINNAMON LEMON AND LIME PRESERVES

Yields: 1 quart

You will need:

- 1 ½ lb. lemons, at room temperature
- 1 ½ lb. limes, at room temperature
- 6 Tbsp. freshly squeezed lemon and/or lime juice, or more if needed
- ½ cup sea salt
- 2 cinnamon sticks

How to Prepare:

Roll the lemons and limes on a table or countertop with your hand. Then, slice each into four wedges and remove the seeds. Set aside.

Sprinkle some of the salt in the clean jar. After that, alternate the layers of lemon and lime wedges with the remaining salt. Pour the lemon or lime juice over everything, making sure that everything is submerged. Ensure that there is an inch of space between the rim of the jar and the surface of the juices.

Once it is ready, seal the jar and place it in a cool, dry shelf away from direct sunlight. For 14 days, open the jar and press down on the preserves to allow the extraction of more juice.

After 14 days, transfer into the refrigerator. Consume within 12 months.

Peach and Lime Chutney

Yields: 1 ½ quarts

You will need:

- 2 ¼ lb. peaches
- 4 to 6 preserved lime wedges
- ½ cup chopped walnuts
- 3 Tbsp. yogurt whey
- ½ Tbsp. peppercorns
- ½ Tbsp. cloves
- ½ Tbsp. cinnamon

How to Prepare:

Slice the peaches into small, bite-sized pieces, discarding the pits. Place the sliced peaches into a bowl. Dice the preserved limes and place into the bowl of peaches.

Add the walnuts, peppercorns, cloves, cinnamon, and yogurt whey. Mix everything well.

Once mixed, place the mixture into a clean jar. Press down on the mixture to release natural juices. Ensure that everything is completely submerged in the liquids. If not, then add just enough non-chlorinated water until the solids are submerged.

Seal the jar tightly and place in a cool, dry shelf away from direct sunlight. Allow to ferment for 3 days. Open and re-seal once a day to release any tightness in the jar as the fermentation process can cause the mixture to expand.

After day 3, transfer the jar of peach and lime chutney into the refrigerator. Consume within 1 month.

Apple Curry Chutney

Yields: 1 ½ quarts

You will need:

- 4 firm apples, such as Golden Delicious, Granny Smith, or Honeycrisp
- ½ cup freshly squeezed lemon juice
- ½ cup kefir
- ¼ cup brown sugar or other sweetener
- 4 tsp. mild curry powder
- 1 tsp. sea salt

How to Prepare:

Remove the core from the apples. Peel the apples and dice then place in a large bowl. Add the lemon juice, kefir, brown sugar, curry powder, and salt and then mix everything well.

Transfer the mixture into a clean jar and cover with a cheesecloth secured with rubber bands. Set on a cool, dry shelf away from direct sunlight and let it ferment for two to four days.

After day 2, taste test the apple curry chutney to check the flavor. If you are satisfied with the balance of sweet and sourness, seal the jar with the lid and refrigerate the chutney for up to 14 days.

Hummus

Yields: 3 cups

You will need:

- 3 cups cooked garbanzo beans
- 3 garlic cloves
- ¼ cup tahini
- ¼ cup freshly squeezed lemon juice
- 3 Tbsp. extra virgin olive oil
- 3 Tbsp. yogurt
- 3 Tbsp. chopped fresh flat leaf parsley
- 1 ½ Tbsp. sea salt
- 1 ½ Tbsp. paprika
- ½ tsp. cumin
- Freshly ground black pepper, to taste

How to Prepare:

Pour the garbanzo beans into a food processor, followed by the tahini, lemon juice, peeled garlic, parsley, yogurt, paprika, sea salt, cumin, and a pinch of black pepper. Cover the food processor and open the smaller lid.

As you process the mixture, gradually pour in the olive oil. Blend everything until smooth and pasty.

Transfer the hummus into a clean container and cover loosely. Set in a cool, dry shelf away from direct sunlight and let it ferment for 8 to 12 hours.

After fermentation, cover the hummus tightly with the lid then refrigerate. Consume within 14 days.

Ginger Ale

Yields: 2 quarts

You will need:

- 2 inches fresh ginger root
- 2 quarts non-chlorinated water
- ¾ cups brown sugar or other sweetener
- ½ cup yogurt whey

How to Prepare:

Peel the ginger and place in a pot with the water. Place over high flame and bring to a boil. Boil for about 5 to 8 minutes to turn the ginger into tea.

Once the green tea is brewed, turn off the heat and stir in the sugar until completely dissolved. Cover and set aside to cool to room temperature.

Once cooled, stir the yogurt whey into the tea and pour into a carboy with an airlock. Place in a cool, dry shelf away from direct sunlight and allow to ferment for 4 to 7 days, or until fizzy.

Once the ginger ale is ready, transfer it into small bottles, leaving some airspace between the cap and the ginger ale. Set aside at room temperature for 5 to 7 days then transfer into the refrigerator. Serve within 6 months.

Kombucha

Yields: 3 quarts

You will need:

- 1 piece SCOBY (Symbiotic Colony of Bacteria and Yeast)
- 3 quarts non-chlorinated water
- 1 ¼ cups kombucha tea, homemade or store-bought
- 1 ¼ cups brown sugar or other sweetener
- 3 tsp loose-leaf green, oolong, or black tea, or 10 grams total in bags

How to Prepare:

Place the tea into a large clean mason jar and set aside.

Pour the water into a small pot, cover, and place over high flame. Once boiling, turn off the flame and pour the freshly boiled water into the jar of tea. Cover and set aside for 15 minutes to steep.

After steeping, strain the tealeaves, or remove the bags. Stir the sugar into the tea using a metal spoon, then seal and set aside at room temperature to cool for about an hour or two.

Once the tea has reached room temperature, stir in half of the kombucha tea and SCOBY. Pour the remaining kombucha tea over the SCOBY and then cover the remaining jar with a cheesecloth secured with rubber bands. Set aside on a warm place away from direct sunlight.

Let the kombucha ferment for up to 5 days, tasting once every day using a clean spoon (do not double-dip!). Once the taste becomes tart instead of sweet, strain the kombucha into a clean jar, seal, and refrigerate. Consume within 6 months. You can use the SCOBY to make a fresh batch of kombucha.

Basic Yogurt

Yields: 1 ½ quarts

You will need:

- ½ cup organic, plain yogurt
- 1 ½ quarts milk

How to Prepare:

Pour the purchased yogurt into a large clean mason jar, or divide them between two smaller mason jars. Set aside.

Pour the milk into a milk pan and place over low flame. Heat to 180 degrees F, or until warm to the touch. Once warmed, dip the bottom of the pan into the basin of ice water to cool down the milk to about 110 degrees F.

Pour the milk into the mason jar/s with the yogurt. Ensure that there is at least an inch of space between the milk and the rim of the jar. Seal the jar/s with its/their lid and shake to mix the milk and yogurt thoroughly.

Place the jar/s of yogurt in a warm place. You can use an incubator or place the jars in a shelf along with some hot water bottles filled with hot water. Allow the yogurt to ferment for up to 24 hours.

Once the yogurt is fermented, transfer into a refrigerator and let it ferment for 1 to 2 weeks.

After two weeks, you may notice that the yogurt is in the lower half of the jar/s while there is cloudy liquid on top. This is called whey and can be strained with a cheesecloth.

To strain the yogurt from the whey, simply rinse and wring out a cheesecloth in non-chlorinated water, then use it to line a strainer. Place the strainer over a bowl and then spoon the yogurt over it.

Allow the yogurt to drain before transferring it into an airtight container. You can also transfer the whey into a separate airtight container. Refrigerate both to store and consume within 6 to 8 weeks.

KEFIR

Yields: 1 ½ quarts

You will need:

- 1 ½ quarts milk

- 3 Tbsp. kefir grains

How to Prepare:

Pour the milk into a milk pan and place over low flame. Heat to 180 degrees F, or until warm to the touch. Once warmed, dip the bottom of the pan into the basin of ice water to quickly cool down the milk to about 110 degrees F.

Transfer the milk into a large clean mason jar or two, ensuring there is at least an inch of headspace between the rim of the jar and the milk. Add the kefir grains, cover, and shake to mix well.

Set the jar/s of milk on a cool, dry shelf for up to 24 hours. Shake once every hour or two. After 12 to 24 hours, shake the mixture one last time and prepare another clean mason jar. Strain the kefir using a strainer lined with a damp cheesecloth and then seal and refrigerate. Consume the kefir within 6 months. You can use the kefir grains in the strainer to make more kefir.

Conclusion

A healthy gut is essential to us in so many ways. Without a healthy gut, we can become susceptible to a range of unpleasant conditions which can manifest themselves in any number of ways and contribute to long term and chronic illnesses. Now you can help to maintain a healthy gut by starting the process of fermenting vegetables and other probiotic foods in the comfort of your own home.

The next step is to start making fermented vegetables!

This simple guide has that you need to know on how to begin, the only thing left to do is to test it. Start small by choosing only one recipe and using the equipment and ingredients you already have lying around in your kitchen. Do not be afraid to make mistakes, because it is all part of the learning process.

As you continue to gain confidence in making your own fermented vegetables, you will eventually discover that it is easy yet beneficial to your digestive health and overall well-being.

Before you go…

I hope you received value from this book and, therefore, I would like to ask you for a favor. Would you be kind enough to leave a review for this book on Amazon?

I want to reach as many people as I can with this book, and more reviews will help me accomplish that and continue writing books that will help people change their lives and get the results they are after.

Thank you for your time and I wish you the best of luck with Fermented Foods!

Sarah Jones

OTHER BOOKS BY SARAH JONES:

Leaky Gut No More. 12 Proven Ways to Heal Leaky Gut Naturally (The Gut Repair Book Series, Book1)

GAPS Diet. 30 Nutrient-Dense Recipes to Alleviate Chronic Inflammation, Repair the Gut Wall and Regain Energy (The Gut Repair Book Series, Book2)

Mindfulness. Simple Techniques You Need to Know to Live in The Moment and Relieve Stress, Anxiety and Depression for Good (Mindfulness Book Series, Book 1)

Mindfulness for Social Anxiety Relief. Learn How to Regain Control of Your Life and Overcome Social Anxiety, Fear, Worry and Self-Criticism Forever (Mindfulness Book Series, Book 2)

Mindful Eating. How to Stop Binge Eating and Overeating, Lose Weight Permanently and Forever Heal Your Relationship with Food (Mindfulness Book Series, Book 3)

Depression. 22 Ways They Don't Want You To Know To Naturally Cure Depression For The Rest Of Your Life

Printed in Great Britain
by Amazon